PELVIC FLOOR EXERCISES

A Detailed Manual On Exercises, Preventative Measures, And Recovery Techniques And Strengthening And Rehabilitating Your Core Muscles

CONTENT

INTRODUCTION

A. Importance of Pelvic Health:

The pelvic floor is a crucial yet often overlooked part of our anatomy. Nestled at the base of the pelvis, this group of muscles plays a pivotal role in supporting the bladder, bowel, and, for women, the uterus. Despite its significance, many people remain unaware of its function until they experience problems.

I. Definition and Function of the Pelvic Floor:

The pelvic floor consists of layers of muscles and tissues stretching like a hammock from the pubic bone at the front to the tailbone at the back. These muscles support the pelvic organs, help maintain continence, and contribute to sexual function. They work in coordination with the abdominal and back muscles to stabilize and support the spine, playing a key role in core strength and overall stability.

II. Common Issues Related to Weak Pelvic Floor Muscles:

A weak pelvic floor can lead to a range of uncomfortable and sometimes debilitating issues. Urinary incontinence, fecal incontinence, and pelvic organ prolapse are among the most common problems. These conditions can significantly impact quality of life, leading to physical discomfort, social embarrassment, and emotional distress. Additionally, weak pelvic floor muscles can contribute to sexual dysfunction, causing pain and reducing sexual satisfaction.

III. Benefits of Strong Pelvic Floor Muscles:

Strengthening the pelvic floor muscles offers numerous benefits. Improved bladder and bowel control, reduced risk of pelvic organ prolapse, and enhanced sexual function are among the primary advantages. For women, strong pelvic floor muscles can facilitate childbirth and promote quicker postpartum recovery. Both men and women can experience better core stability, posture, and overall physical performance. Engaging in regular pelvic floor exercises can lead to a greater sense of physical well-being and confidence.

B. Overview of the Book:

I. Purpose and Goals:

"Pelvic Floor Exercises" is designed to educate and empower readers to take charge of their pelvic health. The primary goal of this book is to provide comprehensive information on the importance of the pelvic floor, identify common issues related to its weakness, and offer practical exercises to strengthen these critical muscles. By the end of this book, readers will have the knowledge and tools necessary to improve their pelvic health, enhance their quality of life, and prevent potential problems.

II. Target Audience:

This book is intended for anyone interested in improving their pelvic health. It is particularly beneficial for individuals experiencing symptoms of pelvic floor weakness, such as incontinence or pelvic pain. Women who are pregnant or postpartum, athletes looking to enhance their core strength, and older adults seeking to maintain their independence and physical function will find this book especially valuable. Healthcare professionals can also use this book as a resource for educating and guiding their patients.

III. Structure of the Book:

The book is structured to provide a logical progression from understanding the basics of the pelvic floor to implementing effective exercises. It begins with a detailed explanation of the anatomy and function of the pelvic floor, followed by a discussion of common issues and their impact on daily life. Subsequent chapters offer a step-by-step guide to pelvic floor exercises, complete with illustrations and tips for proper technique. The book also includes real-life success stories, expert advice, and a section on how to integrate these exercises into a holistic approach to health and fitness.

By delving into the vital topic of pelvic health, "Pelvic Floor Exercises" aims to inspire and guide readers on their journey to stronger, healthier pelvic muscles, and a better quality of life.

UNDERSTANDING THE PELVIC FLOOR

A. Anatomy and Physiology:

I. Detailed Description of Pelvic Floor Muscles:

The pelvic floor is a complex structure composed of muscles, ligaments, and connective tissues that span the area beneath the pelvis. These muscles form a hammock-like support system that holds the pelvic organs, including the bladder, rectum, and for women, the uterus and vagina, in place. The primary muscles of the pelvic floor are:

1. Levator Ani Group: This includes the pubococcygeus, puborectalis, and iliococcygeus muscles. These muscles are critical for maintaining continence and supporting pelvic organs.

Pubococcygeus: This muscle stretches from the pubic bone to the coccyx (tailbone) and controls urine flow and contracts during orgasm.

Puborectalis: Forms a sling around the rectum, playing a key role in maintaining fecal continence.

Iliococcygeus: Supports the pelvic organs and works in tandem with other levator ani muscles.

2. Coccygeus (Ischiococcygeus): This muscle extends from the ischial spine to the sacrum and coccyx, providing additional support to the pelvic organs and stabilizing the sacroiliac joint.

3. Deep Urogenital Diaphragm: Consists of the deep transverse perineal muscle and the sphincter urethrae, these muscles support the urogenital organs and help control the release of urine.

4. Perineal Muscles: Including the bulbospongiosus and ischiocavernosus, these muscles are involved in sexual function and support of the pelvic organs.

II. Interaction with Other Body Systems:

The pelvic floor does not function in isolation; it interacts intricately with various body systems:

Urinary System: The pelvic floor muscles support the bladder and urethra, playing a critical role in urinary continence. Proper functioning of these muscles helps prevent involuntary leakage of urine.

Reproductive System: In women, the pelvic floor muscles support the uterus, vagina, and associated reproductive organs. In men, they support the prostate and play a role in erectile function and ejaculation.

Digestive System: These muscles support the rectum and are crucial for maintaining fecal continence. They work in coordination with the abdominal muscles and diaphragm during defecation.

Musculoskeletal System: The pelvic floor muscles contribute to the stability and mobility of the pelvis and lower back. They work in conjunction with the abdominal and back muscles to maintain posture and support movements.

Nervous System: The pelvic floor is innervated by the pudendal nerve, which controls sensation and muscle contractions. Proper nerve function is essential for maintaining continence and sexual function.

III. Differences Between Male and Female Pelvic Floors:

While the basic structure of the pelvic floor is similar in both sexes, there are notable differences:

Anatomy: In females, the pelvic floor has openings for the urethra, vagina, and rectum, whereas in males, it supports the urethra and rectum. The female pelvic floor also supports the uterus.

Muscle Composition: Women generally have a wider and more elastic pelvic floor to accommodate childbirth, whereas men have a narrower and more stable pelvic floor.

Function: In women, the pelvic floor undergoes significant changes during pregnancy and childbirth, which can affect its function. In men, the pelvic floor muscles are more focused on supporting the prostate and aiding in erectile function.

B. Common Pelvic Floor Disorders:

I. Urinary Incontinence:

Urinary incontinence, the involuntary leakage of urine, is a common pelvic floor disorder affecting both men and women. It can result from weak or damaged pelvic floor muscles, often due to childbirth, surgery, aging, or obesity. There are several types of urinary incontinence:

Stress Incontinence: Leakage occurs during activities that increase abdominal pressure, such as coughing, sneezing, or lifting heavy objects.

Urge Incontinence: A sudden, intense urge to urinate followed by involuntary leakage. Often associated with overactive bladder syndrome.

Mixed Incontinence: A combination of stress and urge incontinence.

Overflow Incontinence: Involuntary leakage due to a full bladder that cannot empty completely.

II. Pelvic Organ Prolapse:

Pelvic organ prolapse occurs when pelvic organs, such as the bladder, uterus, or rectum, descend into or outside of the vaginal canal due to weakened pelvic floor muscles. This condition is more common in women, especially those who have had multiple vaginal deliveries. Types of prolapse include:

Cystocele: Prolapse of the bladder into the vagina.

Rectocele: Prolapse of the rectum into the vagina.

Uterine Prolapse: Descent of the uterus into the vaginal canal.

Enterocele: Prolapse of the small intestine into the vaginal space.

Symptoms include a feeling of pressure or fullness in the pelvis, urinary and bowel difficulties, and discomfort during sexual activity.

III. Sexual Dysfunction:

Pelvic floor disorders can lead to sexual dysfunction in both men and women. In women, weakened or overly tight pelvic floor muscles can cause pain during intercourse (dyspareunia), reduced sensation, and difficulty achieving orgasm. In men, pelvic floor dysfunction can contribute to erectile dysfunction, premature ejaculation, and pain during ejaculation. Addressing pelvic floor health can significantly improve sexual function and overall quality of life.

IV. Chronic Pelvic Pain:

Chronic pelvic pain is a debilitating condition characterized by persistent pain in the pelvic region, lasting six months or longer. It can result from various factors, including pelvic floor muscle tension, endometriosis, interstitial cystitis, and irritable bowel syndrome. Symptoms may include:

Pelvic or lower abdominal pain: Constant or intermittent discomfort.

Pain during urination or bowel movements: Often associated with urinary or digestive issues.

Pain during sexual activity: Can affect both men and women.

Muscle spasms: In the pelvic floor, contributing to pain and discomfort.

Effective management of chronic pelvic pain often involves a multidisciplinary approach, including physical therapy, medication, and lifestyle modifications.

Understanding the anatomy and physiology of the pelvic floor, along with recognizing common disorders, is crucial for maintaining pelvic health and addressing related issues. In the next chapter, we will delve into the importance of pelvic floor exercises and how they can help in preventing and managing these disorders.

BENEFITS OF PELVIC FLOOR EXERCISES

Pelvic floor exercises, often referred to as Kegel exercises, provide numerous benefits for both women and men. These exercises, which involve the repeated contraction and relaxation of the pelvic floor muscles, are a simple yet effective way to enhance physical health and well-being. This chapter delves into the specific benefits of pelvic floor exercises for women and men, highlighting their significance in various stages of life and health conditions.

A. Benefits for Women:

I. Postpartum Recovery:

Childbirth places significant stress on a woman's body, particularly on the pelvic floor muscles. These muscles can become weakened or damaged during delivery, leading to discomfort and various postpartum complications. Engaging in pelvic floor exercises can expedite postpartum recovery by:

Strengthening Muscles: Regularly performing Kegel exercises helps in regaining the strength and tone of the pelvic floor muscles that are stretched during childbirth.

Reducing Discomfort: Strengthened muscles can alleviate discomfort and reduce the likelihood of experiencing pelvic pain.

Supporting Organs: Strong pelvic floor muscles provide better support to the bladder, uterus, and bowels, minimizing the risk of pelvic organ prolapse.

II. Menopause Support:

Menopause brings a host of changes to a woman's body, many of which can affect the pelvic floor. Hormonal fluctuations can lead to a weakening of these muscles, causing issues such as urinary incontinence. Pelvic floor exercises offer essential support during menopause by:

Enhancing Muscle Tone: These exercises help maintain muscle tone, counteracting the natural decline due to hormonal changes.

Preventing Leakage: Improved muscle strength helps in controlling urinary function, reducing episodes of incontinence.

Boosting Confidence: By managing symptoms effectively, women can experience a boost in their confidence and overall quality of life during menopause.

III. Prevention of Urinary Incontinence:

Urinary incontinence is a common issue that can affect women of all ages, often due to weakened pelvic floor muscles. Regularly practicing pelvic floor exercises can play a crucial role in preventing this condition:

Strengthening the Bladder Control Muscles: Consistent exercise helps fortify the muscles responsible for controlling bladder function.

Improving Continence: Stronger pelvic floor muscles improve the ability to hold urine, thus reducing the incidence of accidental leaks.

Enhancing Daily Life: Women can participate more confidently in daily activities, knowing they have better control over their bladder.

B. Benefits for Men:

I. Prostate Health:

Pelvic floor exercises are not just beneficial for women; they also play a vital role in men's health, particularly concerning the prostate. As men age, prostate health can become a concern, and pelvic floor exercises can contribute to maintaining a healthy prostate by:

Supporting Prostate Function: Strong pelvic floor muscles support the prostate and help in maintaining its function.

Aiding Post-Surgery Recovery: For men who undergo prostate surgery, these exercises can aid in faster recovery and help regain control over urinary functions.

Reducing Symptoms: Regular exercise can alleviate symptoms of benign prostatic hyperplasia (BPH) by improving urinary flow and reducing the frequency of urination.

II. Improved Sexual Function:

Men can also experience significant improvements in sexual function through consistent pelvic floor exercises. These benefits include:

Enhanced Erectile Function: Strong pelvic floor muscles can improve blood flow to the penis, leading to stronger and longer-lasting erections.

Increased Control: Better muscle control can lead to improved management of ejaculation, enhancing sexual performance and satisfaction.

Boosted Confidence: With improved sexual function, men often experience a boost in self-esteem and sexual confidence.

III. Prevention of Urinary Incontinence:

Similar to women, men can also suffer from urinary incontinence, especially following prostate surgery or due to aging. Pelvic floor exercises can help prevent this issue by:

Reinforcing Muscle Strength: Regularly exercising the pelvic floor muscles helps maintain their strength and function.

Improving Bladder Control: Enhanced muscle tone provides better control over urinary functions, reducing the risk of incontinence.

Promoting Overall Health: Maintaining strong pelvic floor muscles contributes to better overall health and quality of life.

ASSESSMENT AND PREPARATION

A. Self-Assessment Techniques:

Before beginning any pelvic floor exercise regimen, it is crucial to understand your starting point. Self-assessment techniques help identify your pelvic floor muscle strength and recognize any symptoms of dysfunction.

I. Identifying Pelvic Floor Muscle Strength:

To assess the strength of your pelvic floor muscles, you can try the following techniques:

1. The Stop-Test: One of the simplest methods is to try stopping your urine midstream. While urinating, attempt to halt the flow of urine by contracting your pelvic floor muscles. If you can stop the flow easily, it indicates good muscle strength. However, avoid making this a habit as it can interfere with normal bladder function.

2. Visual Observation: Using a mirror, you can visually observe the contraction of your pelvic floor muscles. Lie down in a comfortable position and place a mirror between your legs. Contract your pelvic floor muscles and look for a visible lift in the perineal area. This lift indicates muscle contraction.

3. Internal Examination: If you feel comfortable, you can insert a clean finger into your vagina or rectum and try to contract your pelvic floor muscles. You should feel a tightening and lifting sensation around your finger. This method provides direct feedback on muscle strength.

4. Kegel Exercises: Perform a Kegel exercise by tightening your pelvic floor muscles as if you were trying to prevent passing gas or stopping the flow of urine. Hold the contraction for a few seconds and then release. Repeat this several times and pay attention to how effectively you can contract and relax the muscles.

II. Recognizing Symptoms of Pelvic Floor Dysfunction:

Recognizing the symptoms of pelvic floor dysfunction is essential to tailor your exercise program appropriately. Common symptoms include:

1. Incontinence: This includes urinary or fecal incontinence, where there is an involuntary leakage of urine or stool.

2. Pelvic Pain: Persistent pain in the pelvic region, including pain during sexual intercourse, can indicate dysfunction.

3. Pressure or Heaviness: A sensation of pressure or heaviness in the pelvic area, sometimes described as a feeling that something is falling out.

4. Frequent Urination: Needing to urinate frequently or experiencing an urgent need to urinate even when the bladder is not full.

5. Incomplete Emptying: Feeling like the bladder or bowel is not completely empty after using the restroom.

If you identify any of these symptoms, it may be indicative of pelvic floor dysfunction and warrant further evaluation.

B. Professional Assessments:

While self-assessment is a good starting point, professional assessments provide a comprehensive evaluation of your pelvic floor health. Understanding when to seek help and the types of clinical evaluations available can guide you in your journey.

I. When to See a Healthcare Provider:

Consider consulting a healthcare provider if:

1. Persistent Symptoms: You have persistent symptoms of pelvic floor dysfunction that do not improve with self-care.

2. Uncertain Diagnosis: You are unsure about your symptoms or cannot accurately assess your pelvic floor muscle strength.

3. Specialized Advice: You need specialized advice or treatment options that are beyond self-assessment and basic exercises.

4. Post-Surgery or Childbirth: If you have recently undergone pelvic surgery or childbirth, professional assessment is crucial to determine the appropriate recovery exercises.

II. Types of Clinical Evaluations:

Healthcare providers use various methods to evaluate pelvic floor health:

1. Physical Examination: A physical examination by a healthcare provider involves both external and internal assessments to evaluate muscle strength, tone, and any signs of dysfunction.

2. Ultrasound: Ultrasound imaging can visualize the pelvic floor muscles in action, providing detailed information about their function and structure.

3. Pelvic Floor Manometry: This test measures the pressure inside the pelvic floor muscles, helping to assess their strength and endurance.

4. MRI or CT Scan: In some cases, imaging studies like MRI or CT scans may be recommended to get a detailed view of the pelvic anatomy.

5. Biofeedback: Biofeedback involves using sensors to provide real-time feedback on muscle activity, helping you learn how to control and strengthen your pelvic floor muscles effectively.

C. Preparing for Exercise:

Proper preparation is key to a successful pelvic floor exercise regimen. Setting clear goals, having the necessary equipment, and creating a conducive environment will enhance your exercise experience.

I. Setting Goals and Expectations:

Before starting, it is essential to set realistic goals and expectations. Determine what you want to achieve with pelvic floor exercises. Goals can include:

1. Improving Muscle Strength: Aim to strengthen the pelvic floor muscles to prevent or reduce symptoms of dysfunction.

2. Enhancing Bladder Control: Work towards better bladder control and reducing incidents of incontinence.

3. Reducing Pain: Aim to alleviate pelvic pain and discomfort through targeted exercises.

4. Postpartum Recovery: Focus on restoring pelvic floor function after childbirth.

Having clear goals will help you stay motivated and track your progress.

II. Necessary Equipment and Attire:

While pelvic floor exercises typically do not require special equipment, some tools can enhance your workout:

1. Exercise Mat: A comfortable mat provides support during floor exercises.

2. Kegel Weights: These weights, also known as vaginal weights or cones, can be used to add resistance to Kegel exercises, increasing their effectiveness.

3. Biofeedback Devices: These devices provide feedback on muscle activity, helping you perform exercises correctly.

4. Comfortable Clothing: Wear loose, comfortable clothing that allows for a full range of motion.

III. Creating a Conducive Environment:

Establishing a conducive environment for your exercises can significantly impact your consistency and success:

1. Quiet Space: Find a quiet and private space where you can focus without interruptions.

2. Regular Schedule: Set a regular time for your exercises to build a routine and ensure consistency.

3. Mindfulness and Relaxation: Incorporate mindfulness techniques and relaxation exercises to enhance the connection with your pelvic floor muscles.

4. Support System: If possible, involve a partner or friend who can provide support and motivation.

By following these steps, you can effectively prepare for your pelvic floor exercise regimen, setting a strong foundation for improved pelvic health.

BASIC PELVIC FLOOR EXERCISES

In this chapter, we will delve into some of the most effective exercises for strengthening the pelvic floor muscles. These exercises not only improve pelvic health but also enhance overall well-being. We'll cover Kegel exercises, the bridge pose, and squats, providing historical context, step-by-step guides, and tips to avoid common mistakes. Let's begin our journey to a stronger, healthier pelvic floor.

A. Kegel Exercises:

I. History and Development:

Kegel exercises, named after Dr. Arnold Kegel, who first described them in the 1940s, were initially developed to help women who experienced urinary incontinence post-childbirth. Dr. Kegel discovered that by strengthening the pelvic floor muscles, patients could gain better control over their bladder and improve overall pelvic health. Over time, Kegel exercises have become a cornerstone in treating various pelvic floor dysfunctions, benefiting both men and women.

II. Step-by-Step Guide:

1. Identify the Pelvic Floor Muscles: The easiest way to locate these muscles is by trying to stop the flow of urine midstream. The muscles you use are your pelvic floor muscles.

2. Find a Comfortable Position: You can do Kegel exercises sitting, standing, or lying down. Beginners may find it easiest to start lying down.

3. Contract the Muscles: Tighten your pelvic floor muscles and hold the contraction for 3-5 seconds.

4. Release: Relax the muscles completely for 3-5 seconds.

5. Repeat: Aim for 10-15 repetitions per session, gradually increasing the hold time as

your muscles get stronger. Perform this exercise 3 times a day.

III. Common Mistakes to Avoid:

1. Using the Wrong Muscles: Ensure you're not contracting your abdomen, thighs, or buttocks. Focus solely on the pelvic floor muscles.

2. Overdoing It: More isn't always better. Overworking the muscles can lead to fatigue and diminish the benefits.

3. Holding Your Breath: Remember to breathe normally during the exercises. Holding your breath can increase abdominal pressure and reduce the effectiveness.

B. Bridge Pose:

I. Benefits and Execution:

Benefits: The bridge pose, or Setu Bandhasana, is a yoga posture that strengthens the pelvic floor, glutes, and lower back muscles. It also improves spinal flexibility and can alleviate back pain.

Execution:

1. Start Position: Lie on your back with your knees bent and feet flat on the floor, hip-width apart. Place your arms alongside your body with palms facing down.

2. Lift the Hips: Press your feet into the ground as you lift your hips towards the ceiling. Engage your core and pelvic floor muscles.

3. Hold: Hold the position for 5-10 seconds, keeping your thighs parallel and avoiding overarching your back.

4. Lower: Slowly lower your hips back to the floor. Repeat the movement 10-15 times.

II. Variations for Different Fitness Levels:

1. Beginner: Place a block or pillow under your lower back for support, reducing the range of motion.

2. Intermediate: Perform the bridge with one leg lifted, keeping the other leg bent and foot on the floor. Alternate legs with each repetition.

3. Advanced: Try a full wheel pose (Urdhva Dhanurasana) for a deeper stretch and greater challenge to the pelvic floor and core muscles.

C. Squats:

I. Importance for Pelvic Strength:

Squats are fundamental exercises that target multiple muscle groups, including the pelvic floor, glutes, quadriceps, and hamstrings. They enhance lower body strength, improve balance, and support pelvic health by engaging the pelvic floor muscles.

II. Proper Technique and Modifications:

Proper Technique:

1. Start Position: Stand with your feet shoulder-width apart, toes pointing slightly outward.

2. Lowering: Push your hips back and bend your knees to lower your body as if sitting into a chair. Keep your chest lifted and spine neutral.

3. Depth: Lower down until your thighs are parallel to the floor or as far as your flexibility allows.

4. Rising: Press through your heels to return to the starting position. Squeeze your glutes at the top and engage your pelvic floor muscles.

5. Repetitions: Aim for 3 sets of 10-15 repetitions, adjusting based on your fitness level.

Modifications:

1. Beginner: Use a chair for support. Sit down and stand up from the chair, focusing on engaging your pelvic floor muscles.

2. Intermediate: Hold a weight (such as a dumbbell or kettlebell) close to your chest to add resistance.

3. Advanced: Perform jump squats, adding a plyometric element to increase intensity and engage your pelvic floor muscles more dynamically.

ADVANCED PELVIC FLOOR EXERCISES

As you progress in your pelvic floor training, it's important to move beyond the basics and incorporate more advanced exercises that not only strengthen your pelvic floor but also enhance overall core stability, flexibility, and mindfulness. This chapter focuses on three key areas: Pelvic Tilts, Core Integration, and the incorporation of Yoga and Pilates into your routine.

A. Pelvic Tilts:

I. Technique and Benefits:

Pelvic tilts are a fundamental exercise that helps to mobilize the lower spine and pelvis, improveposture, and strengthen the pelvic floor muscles. Here's how to perform pelvic tilts correctly:

1. Starting Position: Lie on your back with your knees bent, feet flat on the floor, and arms at your sides. Ensure your spine is in a

neutral position, with a small natural curve in your lower back.

2. Execution:

Inhale deeply to prepare.

As you exhale, gently tilt your pelvis backward, pressing your lower back into the floor. Engage your abdominal muscles and pelvic floor as you do this.

Hold the tilt for a few seconds while maintaining your breath.

Inhale and return to the starting position, allowing your lower back to arch slightly off the floor.

Repeat for 10-15 repetitions, focusing on controlled and smooth movements.

Benefits:

Strengthens the pelvic floor: By engaging the pelvic muscles, pelvic tilts help to improve their strength and endurance.

Enhances core stability: This exercise activates the abdominal muscles, promoting better core stability.

Improves posture: Regular practice can correct postural imbalances by aligning the pelvis and spine.

Reduces lower back pain: Mobilizing the lumbar spine can alleviate discomfort and tension in the lower back.

II. Incorporating into Daily Routine:

Incorporating pelvic tilts into your daily routine is straightforward and can be done almost anywhere:

Morning Routine: Start your day with a few sets of pelvic tilts to wake up your core and pelvic floor.

Work Breaks: If you have a sedentary job, take breaks to perform pelvic tilts while seated or standing to keep your pelvic muscles active.

Pre-Bedtime Routine: Wind down with gentle pelvic tilts to relax your lower back and pelvic muscles before sleeping.

B. Core Integration:

I. Connecting Core Strength to Pelvic Health:

A strong core is crucial for pelvic health, as the muscles of the abdomen, back, and pelvic floor work synergistically to provide stability and support. By integrating core exercises into your routine, you can enhance the effectiveness of your pelvic floor training.

II. Exercises like Planks and Leg Raises:

Planks:

Technique:

Start in a forearm plank position with elbows directly under your shoulders and your body in a straight line from head to heels.

Engage your core, glutes, and pelvic floor to maintain the position.

Hold for 20-30 seconds, gradually increasing the duration as your strength improves.

Benefits:

Full-body engagement: Planks work not only the core but also the shoulders, back, and legs.

Pelvic floor activation: Maintaining a plank requires the engagement of the pelvic floor muscles.

Improves endurance: Holding the plank position builds muscular endurance.

Leg Raises:

Technique:

Lie on your back with your legs extended straight.

Place your hands under your hips for support.

Slowly lift your legs towards the ceiling while keeping them straight.

Lower them back down without touching the floor.

Perform 10-15 repetitions.

Benefits:

Strengthens lower abs: Leg raises target the lower abdominal muscles, which support the pelvic floor.

Enhances coordination: This exercise requires control and coordination, benefiting overall muscle function.

Improves pelvic stability: The pelvic floor muscles are activated to stabilize the pelvis during leg raises.

C. Yoga and Pilates:

I. Specific Poses and Routines:

Yoga:

Bridge Pose (Setu Bandhasana): Strengthens the glutes, lower back, and pelvic floor.

Lie on your back with your knees bent and feet hip-width apart.

Press into your feet to lift your hips, engaging your glutes and pelvic floor.

Hold for 20-30 seconds, then lower back down.

Child's Pose (Balasana): Stretches the lower back and relaxes the pelvic floor.

Kneel on the floor, sit back on your heels, and extend your arms forward.

Rest your forehead on the ground and breathe deeply.

Pilates:

Pelvic Curl: Similar to pelvic tilts but performed in a flowing motion.

 Lie on your back with knees bent and feet flat.

Roll your spine off the floor, lifting your hips towards the ceiling.

Lower back down one vertebra at a time.

Hundred: Enhances core strength and stability.

Lie on your back with your legs in a tabletop position.

Lift your head, neck, and shoulders off the floor.

Pump your arms up and down for a count of 100, keeping your core and pelvic floor engaged.

II. Focus on Breath and Mindfulness:

Breath control and mindfulness are integral to both Yoga and Pilates, and they significantly enhance pelvic floor training:

Breath Control: Proper breathing techniques ensure that the pelvic floor muscles work in harmony with the diaphragm and abdominal muscles. Inhale deeply to expand your diaphragm and exhale fully to engage your core and pelvic floor.

Mindfulness: Being present during your exercises helps you to connect with your body, recognize tension, and ensure proper form. This awareness leads to more effective and safer workouts.

By integrating advanced pelvic floor exercises into your routine, you can achieve a stronger, more stable core, improve your overall health, and enhance your quality of life. Remember to progress at your own pace, listen to your body, and stay consistent with your practice.

PELVIC FLOOR EXERCISES FOR SPECIFIC CONDITIONS

Pelvic floor exercises are vital for maintaining and improving the health of the pelvic region. This chapter focuses on tailored pelvic floor exercise programs for specific conditions, including postpartum recovery, menopausal support, and chronic pain management. Each section outlines safe, effective, and progressive exercise plans to address the unique needs of individuals experiencing these conditions.

A. Postpartum Recovery:

Pregnancy and childbirth can significantly impact the pelvic floor muscles. Postpartum recovery is crucial for new mothers to regain strength, prevent incontinence, and support overall pelvic health. This section provides safe exercises and a gradual progression plan for postpartum recovery.

I. Safe Exercises for New Mothers:

In the initial weeks postpartum, it's essential to begin with gentle exercises that do not strain the pelvic floor. The following exercises are safe and effective for new mothers:

1. Pelvic Tilts: Lie on your back with knees bent and feet flat on the floor. Gently tilt your pelvis upward, tightening your abdominal muscles. Hold for a few seconds and release. Repeat 10 times.

2. Kegel Exercises: Contract and relax the pelvic floor muscles as if you are stopping the flow of urine. Hold the contraction for 3-5 seconds and release. Repeat 10-15 times, gradually increasing the duration of the hold as you gain strength.

3. Bridge Pose: Lie on your back with knees bent and feet flat on the floor. Lift your hips toward the ceiling, engaging your glutes and pelvic floor. Hold for a few seconds and slowly lower down. Repeat 10 times.

4. Transverse Abdominis Activation: While lying on your back, place your hands on your lower abdomen. Inhale deeply, then exhale and draw your belly button toward your spine. Hold for a few seconds and release. Repeat 10 times.

II. Gradual Progression Plan:

As your body heals and strengthens, it's important to gradually increase the intensity and variety of exercises. The following plan provides a progressive approach to postpartum pelvic floor recovery:

1. Weeks 1-4: Focus on gentle pelvic tilts, Kegel exercises, and transverse abdominis activation. Aim for two sets of each exercise daily.

2. Weeks 5-8: Introduce bridge poses and increase the duration and intensity of Kegel exercises. Perform three sets of each exercise, three times a week.

3. Months 3-6: Add squats and lunges to your routine to further strengthen the pelvic floor and surrounding muscles. Perform three sets of each exercise, four times a week.

4. Beyond 6 Months: Continue with a balanced exercise routine that includes pelvic floor exercises, core strengthening, and overall body conditioning. Aim for a minimum of three sessions per week.

B. Menopausal Support:

Menopause brings hormonal changes that can affect the pelvic floor, leading to symptoms such as incontinence and pelvic discomfort. Tailored exercises can help manage these symptoms and support pelvic health during this transition.

I. Tailored Exercises for Hormonal Changes:

Hormonal changes during menopause can lead to the weakening of pelvic floor muscles. The following exercises are designed to counteract these effects:

1. Deep Breathing with Pelvic Floor Engagement: Sit or lie down in a comfortable position. Inhale deeply, expanding your diaphragm. As you exhale, gently engage your pelvic floor muscles. Repeat 10 times.

2. Pelvic Clocks: Lie on your back with knees bent and feet flat on the floor. Imagine your pelvis is a clock. Gently tilt your pelvis in all directions, moving from 12 o'clock to 6 o'clock, then 3 o'clock to 9 o'clock. This helps improve pelvic mobility and muscle awareness. Repeat for 1-2 minutes.

3. Standing Kegels: Perform Kegel exercises while standing to simulate real-life situations where pelvic floor strength is needed. Hold each contraction for 5-10 seconds and repeat 10-15 times.

II. Managing Symptoms Through Pelvic Health:

Regular pelvic floor exercises can help manage menopausal symptoms such as incontinence and pelvic discomfort. Here are some strategies:

1.   Consistency: Incorporate   pelvic   floor exercises into your daily routine. Consistency is key to maintaining strength and managing symptoms.

2. Combination Exercises: Combine Kegels with other exercises such as squats or lunges to strengthen the pelvic floor and lower body simultaneously.

3.   Relaxation   Techniques: Incorporate relaxation   techniques   such   as   yoga   or meditation   to   reduce   stress,   which   can exacerbate menopausal symptoms.

C. Chronic Pain Management:

Chronic pelvic pain can significantly impact quality of life. Gentle pelvic floor exercises can provide relief and improve function without aggravating   pain.   This   section   outlines exercises and techniques to manage chronic pain.

I. Gentle Exercises for Pain Relief:

For individuals with chronic pelvic pain, gentle exercises that do not increase discomfort are crucial. The following exercises can help alleviate pain:

1. Child's Pose: Kneel on the floor, sit back on your heels, and stretch your arms forward, resting your forehead on the ground. Hold this position for 1-2 minutes, breathing deeply to relax the pelvic floor.

2. Pelvic Floor Drop: Sit comfortably on a chair or exercise ball. Inhale deeply, allowing your pelvic floor to relax and "drop." Exhale and gently contract your pelvic floor. Repeat 10 times, focusing on relaxation.

3. Happy Baby Pose: Lie on your back, bend your knees, and bring them toward your chest. Hold the outside of your feet with your hands and gently pull your knees toward the floor. Hold for 1-2 minutes, breathing deeply to release tension.

II. Techniques to Avoid Aggravating Pain:

It's important to avoid exercises and techniques that could aggravate chronic pelvic pain. Here are some tips:

1. Avoid High-Impact Activities: Activities such as running or jumping can increase pelvic floor stress. Opt for low-impact exercises like swimming or cycling.

2. Gradual Progression: Increase the intensity and duration of exercises gradually to avoid overloading the pelvic floor.

3. Listen to Your Body: Pay attention to your body's signals. If an exercise causes pain, stop and try a gentler alternative.

4. Professional Guidance: Consider consulting a physical therapist specialized in pelvic floor health to develop a personalized exercise plan that addresses your specific needs.

PELVIC FLOOR EXERCISES FOR SPECIFIC CONDITIONS

Pelvic floor exercises offer tailored solutions for a range of conditions. In this chapter, we explore how these exercises can aid in postpartum recovery, support menopausal health, and manage chronic pain.

A. Postpartum Recovery:

The postpartum period is a crucial time for new mothers to focus on restoring their pelvic floor strength and overall well-being. Pregnancy and childbirth can significantly weaken the pelvic muscles, leading to issues such as incontinence and pelvic organ prolapse. Implementing a safe and gradual exercise plan can help new mothers recover effectively.

I. Safe Exercises for New Mothers:

1. Kegel Exercises: These are fundamental exercises that involve contracting and relaxing the pelvic floor muscles. To perform a Kegel:

Sit or lie down comfortably.

Tighten the muscles you use to stop urination.

Hold for a count of five, then relax for five seconds.

Repeat 10 times, three times a day.

2. Pelvic Tilts: These exercises help to gently engage and strengthen the core and pelvic floor muscles.

Lie on your back with knees bent and feet flat on the floor.

Inhale deeply, then as you exhale, tilt your pelvis upward, flattening your lower back against the floor.

Hold for a few seconds, then release.

Perform 10 repetitions.

3. Bridge Exercise: This exercise targets the glutes and the pelvic floor.

Lie on your back with knees bent and feet hip-width apart.

Press through your heels to lift your hips off the floor, squeezing your glutes.

Hold for a few seconds at the top, then lower back down.

Repeat 10-15 times.

II. Gradual Progression Plan:

A gradual progression plan is essential to avoid overexertion and ensure a safe recovery. Here's a suggested plan for postpartum mothers:

1. Weeks 1-2:

Focus on basic Kegel exercises and gentle pelvic tilts.

Perform these exercises while lying down or sitting to minimize strain.

2. Weeks 3-4:

Continue with Kegels and pelvic tilts, adding in bridge exercises.

Gradually increase the number of repetitions and hold times.

3. Weeks 5-6 and Beyond:

Introduce more advanced pelvic floor exercises, such as squats and lunges.

Begin incorporating light aerobic activities like walking or swimming.

Consistency and patience are key. New mothers should consult with their healthcare provider before starting any exercise program, especially if they have had a complicated delivery.

B. Menopausal Support:

Menopause brings hormonal changes that can impact pelvic health, leading to symptoms like vaginal dryness, urinary incontinence, and pelvic discomfort. Tailored pelvic floor exercises can help manage these symptoms and improve overall quality of life.

I. Tailored Exercises for Hormonal Changes:

1. Deep Breathing with Pelvic Floor Engagement:

Sit comfortably and inhale deeply, allowing your belly to expand.

As you exhale, gently contract your pelvic floor muscles.

Hold for a few seconds, then release and repeat.

2. Wall Squats:

Stand with your back against a wall and feet shoulder-width apart.

Slide down the wall into a squat position, keeping your knees aligned with your toes.

Engage your pelvic floor as you hold the squat for a few seconds.

Return to the starting position and repeat.

3. Yoga for Pelvic Health:

Poses like the Bridge Pose (Setu Bandhasana) and Child's Pose (Balasana) can help stretch and strengthen the pelvic floor.

Practicing these poses regularly can alleviate tension and promote relaxation.

II. Managing Symptoms Through Pelvic Health:

1. Regular Routine:

Incorporate pelvic floor exercises into your daily routine to maintain muscle strength and flexibility.

Aim for at least 10 minutes of focused exercises each day.

2. Hydration and Nutrition:

Staying hydrated and consuming a balanced diet rich in phytoestrogens (found in soy products) can support hormonal balance and pelvic health.

3. Stress Management:

Practice relaxation techniques like meditation or deep breathing to reduce stress, which can exacerbate menopausal symptoms.

4. Consultation with Healthcare Providers:

Regular check-ups with healthcare providers can help monitor progress and adjust exercise routines as needed.

C. Chronic Pain Management:

Chronic pelvic pain can be debilitating, but gentle pelvic floor exercises can provide relief and improve function. It's important to focus on exercises that alleviate pain without causing further discomfort.

I. Gentle Exercises for Pain Relief:

1. Pelvic Floor Relaxation:

Lie on your back with knees bent.

Take deep breaths, focusing on relaxing your pelvic floor muscles with each exhale.

Perform this exercise for 5-10 minutes daily.

2. Leg Drops:

Lie on your back with knees bent and feet flat on the floor.

Slowly lower one leg to the side, keeping the other knee bent.

Return to the starting position and repeat with the other leg.

Perform 10 repetitions on each side.

3. Hip Rolls:

Lie on your back with knees bent and feet flat on the floor.

Gently rock your hips side to side, keeping your upper body relaxed.

Repeat for 1-2 minutes.

II. Techniques to Avoid Aggravating Pain:

1. Listen to Your Body:

Avoid exercises that cause pain or discomfort.

Modify movements as needed to stay within a pain-free range of motion.

2. Gradual Progression:

Start with gentle exercises and gradually increase intensity and duration.

Allow ample time for rest and recovery between sessions.

3. Proper Posture:

Maintain good posture during exercises to avoid unnecessary strain on the pelvic floor.

Focus on aligning your spine and pelvis correctly.

4. Consult a Physical Therapist:

Working with a pelvic floor physical therapist can provide personalized guidance and ensure exercises are performed correctly.

A therapist can also suggest additional pain management techniques, such as biofeedback or manual therapy.

Pelvic floor exercises offer significant benefits for various conditions, from postpartum recovery and menopausal support to chronic pain management. By following tailored exercise plans and consulting healthcare providers, individuals can improve their pelvic health and overall well-being.

INTEGRATING PELVIC FLOOR EXERCISES INTO DAILY LIFE

Pelvic floor exercises are essential for maintaining a healthy and functional pelvic region, but their benefits are maximized when integrated into daily life. This chapter will guide you through developing a routine, incorporating these exercises into other fitness activities, and leveraging mindfulness and relaxation techniques to enhance pelvic health.

A. Developing a Routine:

Building a consistent routine is the cornerstone of effective pelvic floor exercise. Here's how to establish a regimen that seamlessly fits into your daily life.

I. Scheduling and Consistency Tips:

1. Set a Specific Time:

Identify a time of day that you can consistently dedicate to your pelvic floor exercises. This might be first thing in the morning, during your lunch break, or just before bed. Consistency is key, so choose a time when you are least likely to be interrupted.

2. Use Reminders:

Set reminders on your phone or use a habit-tracking app to keep yourself on track. Visual cues, like sticky notes on your mirror or desk, can also serve as effective reminders.

3. Start Small:

Begin with a manageable duration, such as five to ten minutes per day. Gradually increase the time as the exercises become a more ingrained part of your routine.

4. Integrate with Daily Activities:

Incorporate exercises into daily tasks. Perform pelvic floor contractions while brushing your teeth, waiting for your coffee to brew, or during your commute (if you're not driving).

Linking exercises to routine activities helps make them a natural part of your day.

5. Consistency Over Intensity:

Focus on consistency rather than intensity, especially when starting. Regular practice is more beneficial than sporadic, intense sessions.

II. Combining with Other Fitness Activities:

1. Pair with Core Workouts:

Pelvic floor exercises complement core workouts like Pilates and yoga. These disciplines often include movements that engage the pelvic floor, making it easier to incorporate targeted exercises seamlessly.

2. Incorporate into Cardio Sessions:

Engage your pelvic floor muscles during low-impact cardio activities like walking, cycling, or swimming. For example, while walking, focus on contracting and relaxing your pelvic floor muscles in rhythm with your steps.

3. Use Fitness Classes:

Many fitness classes, especially those focused on core strength, can incorporate pelvic floor exercises. Speak to your instructor about your goals and ask if they can suggest specific modifications or additions to your routine.

4. Strength Training Integration:

When lifting weights or performing resistance exercises, activate your pelvic floor muscles to provide stability and support. This not only enhances your pelvic health but also improves overall strength and posture.

B. Mindfulness and Relaxation:

Stress reduction and mindfulness play significant roles in maintaining and improving pelvic health. Here's how to incorporate these elements into your routine.

I. Role of Stress Reduction in Pelvic Health:

1. Understanding the Connection:

Stress and anxiety can lead to muscle tension, including in the pelvic floor. Chronic tension can cause discomfort, pain, and dysfunction. Reducing stress helps relax these muscles and promotes overall pelvic health.

2. Daily Stress Management:

Incorporate stress management techniques into your daily life. Regular exercise, adequate sleep, and healthy eating habits contribute to lower stress levels, indirectly benefiting pelvic health.

II. Techniques like Meditation and Deep Breathing:

1. Meditation:

Regular meditation helps calm the mind and reduce stress. Even a few minutes of meditation each day can significantly impact your overall well-being. Find a quiet space, sit comfortably, and focus on your breath or a mantra. Apps like Headspace or Calm can provide guided sessions to help you get started.

2. Deep Breathing Exercises:

Deep breathing promotes relaxation and can be particularly beneficial for the pelvic floor. Practice diaphragmatic breathing, where you breathe deeply into your abdomen rather than shallow breaths into your chest. Here's a simple exercise:

Sit or lie down in a comfortable position.

Place one hand on your chest and the other on your abdomen.

Inhale deeply through your nose, allowing your abdomen to rise while keeping your chest relatively still.

Exhale slowly through your mouth, letting your abdomen fall.

Repeat for five to ten minutes daily.

3. Progressive Muscle Relaxation:

This technique involves tensing and then relaxing different muscle groups, including the pelvic floor. Starting from your toes, work your way up, tensing each muscle group for a few seconds before releasing. This helps identify and alleviate tension throughout your body.

4. Yoga and Stretching:

Yoga combines physical postures with mindfulness and breathing techniques, making it an excellent practice for pelvic health. Focus on poses that stretch and strengthen the pelvic area, such as Child's Pose, Bridge Pose, and Happy Baby Pose.

Integrating pelvic floor exercises into your daily routine and combining them with mindfulness and relaxation techniques will enhance their effectiveness and contribute to your overall well-being. Remember, the goal is consistency and a holistic approach to pelvic health, making these exercises a natural and enjoyable part of your everyday life.

OVERCOMING CHALLENGES

Embarking on a journey to strengthen the pelvic floor can be empowering and transformative. However, as with any fitness regimen, it comes with its own set of challenges. This chapter will explore common obstacles faced by those who practice pelvic floor exercises and offer strategies for overcoming them. Additionally, we'll delve into the importance of seeking support to maintain motivation and achieve your goals.

A. Common Obstacles:

I. Motivation and Adherence Issues:

One of the most significant challenges in any exercise program is maintaining motivation and adherence. Pelvic floor exercises are no exception. Many people start with enthusiasm but find it difficult to stay committed over time. Several factors contribute to this struggle:

1. Lack of Immediate Results: Unlike more visible forms of exercise, the benefits of pelvic floor exercises may not be immediately apparent. This can lead to frustration and decreased motivation.

2. Monotony: Repetitive routines can become monotonous, making it hard to stay engaged.

3. Busy Schedules: Finding time for a consistent exercise routine can be challenging amidst daily responsibilities and commitments.

Strategies to Overcome Motivation and Adherence Issues:

Set Clear Goals: Define specific, measurable, achievable, relevant, and time-bound (SMART) goals. Whether it's reducing incontinence episodes, improving sexual health, or simply increasing strength, having clear objectives can boost motivation.

Track Progress: Keep a journal or use an app to record your exercises and any improvements you notice. Seeing progress, no matter how small, can be incredibly motivating.

Incorporate Variety: Mix up your routine with different types of pelvic floor exercises to keep things interesting. Combine Kegels with other core-strengthening activities like Pilates or yoga.

Schedule Exercise Time: Treat your exercise time as an important appointment. Consistency is key, so find a time of day that works best for you and stick to it.

II. Physical Limitations and Adaptations:

Physical limitations can also pose significant challenges to those wanting to engage in pelvic floor exercises. These limitations can stem from various conditions, such as chronic pain, recent surgery, or mobility issues.

Adapting Exercises for Physical Limitations:

Consult a Professional: Before starting any exercise program, it's crucial to consult with a healthcare provider or physiotherapist. They can help tailor exercises to your specific needs and limitations.

Start Slow: Begin with gentle exercises and gradually increase intensity as your strength and confidence grow.

Use Props and Modifications: Incorporate props like exercise balls or resistance bands to assist with certain movements. Modifying positions can also make exercises more comfortable and accessible.

Listen to Your Body: Pay close attention to how your body responds to exercises. If something doesn't feel right, stop and seek professional advice.

B. Seeking Support:

Support can be a critical factor in overcoming challenges and achieving long-term success with pelvic floor exercises. Having the right support system can provide encouragement, accountability, and guidance.

I. Finding a Workout Buddy or Support Group:

Having a workout buddy or joining a support group can significantly enhance your exercise experience. The benefits of social support include increased motivation, accountability, and shared experiences.

Benefits of a Workout Buddy:

Motivation: A workout buddy can provide the motivation to stick with your exercise routine, especially on days when you're feeling less inclined to exercise.

Accountability: Knowing that someone else is counting on you can help you stay committed to your regimen.

Shared Experiences: Sharing experiences with someone who understands your challenges can be comforting and encouraging.

Finding a Support Group:

Local Community Centers: Check local community centers or gyms for support groups or exercise classes focused on pelvic floor health.

Online Communities: Numerous online forums and social media groups are dedicated to pelvic floor health. These can be excellent resources for finding support and information.

II. Professional Guidance from Physiotherapists:

Seeking professional guidance from physiotherapists who specialize in pelvic floor health can be invaluable. They can provide personalized exercise plans, monitor your progress, and ensure you're performing exercises correctly.

Benefits of Professional Guidance:

Expert Advice: Physiotherapists have specialized knowledge and can offer tailored advice and exercises based on your individual needs.

Proper Technique: Ensuring you're performing exercises correctly can prevent injury and enhance effectiveness.

Progress Monitoring: Regular check-ins with a physiotherapist can help track your progress and make necessary adjustments to your exercise plan.

How to Find a Qualified Physiotherapist:

Referrals: Ask your primary care provider for a referral to a qualified physiotherapist.

Professional Associations: Check professional associations for certified physiotherapists specializing in pelvic floor health.

Online Directories: Use online directories to find physiotherapists in your area with good reviews and ratings.

TRACKING PROGRESS AND SUCCESS STORIES

Embarking on the journey of pelvic floor exercises is a significant step toward improving your health and well-being. To ensure that your efforts are effective and that you stay motivated, tracking your progress is crucial. This chapter will guide you on how to monitor improvements effectively and share inspiring success stories to keep you motivated.

A. Monitoring Improvements:

Monitoring your progress involves setting clear milestones, using tools and apps, and regularly evaluating your improvements. This process not only keeps you accountable but also allows you to celebrate your successes, no matter how small.

I. Setting Milestones and Goals:

Setting milestones and goals is the first step in tracking your progress. Here are some strategies to help you define and achieve your objectives:

1. Define Clear Goals: Start by identifying what you want to achieve with your pelvic floor exercises. Your goals could range from reducing incontinence, improving sexual health, to enhancing overall pelvic strength. Be specific about your objectives to make them measurable.

2. Set Realistic Milestones: Break down your larger goals into smaller, manageable milestones. For example, if your goal is to improve continence, a milestone could be reducing leakage incidents from daily to once a week. Setting achievable milestones keeps you motivated and focused.

3. Create a Timeline: Establish a timeline for achieving your milestones. This helps you stay on track and gives you a sense of urgency. Ensure that your timeline is realistic, allowing enough time for gradual improvement.

4. Regular Check-Ins: Schedule regular check-ins to assess your progress. These could be

weekly or monthly, depending on your goals. During these check-ins, review your milestones and adjust your plan if needed.

II. Tools and Apps for Tracking:

With technology at our fingertips, there are numerous tools and apps designed to help you track your progress effectively. Here are some of the best options:

1. Fitness Trackers: Devices like Fitbit or Apple Watch can be programmed to remind you to do your exercises and log your activity. They offer features like goal setting, progress tracking, and reminders.

2. Pelvic Floor Exercise Apps: There are several apps specifically designed for pelvic floor exercises, such as Kegel Trainer and Elvie Trainer. These apps guide you through exercises, track your progress, and provide feedback.

3. Journals and Diaries: For those who prefer a more traditional approach, maintaining a

journal or diary can be very effective. Record your daily exercises, any symptoms, and improvements. This manual tracking method helps you stay connected to your progress.

4. Spreadsheets: Creating a spreadsheet to log your exercises and improvements can be an effective tracking tool. You can customize it to your needs and easily visualize your progress with charts and graphs.

B. Real-Life Success Stories:

Success stories from others who have undertaken similar journeys can be incredibly motivating. These testimonials and case studies offer valuable insights and lessons that can inspire and guide you.

I. Testimonials and Case Studies:

1. Mary's Journey to Continence: Mary, a 45-year-old mother of two, struggled with incontinence for years. After committing to a pelvic floor exercise routine and using a tracking app, she saw significant

improvements within six months. Mary's dedication and consistent effort paid off, and she now enjoys a life free from incontinence.

2. John's Road to Recovery: John, a 50-year-old who underwent prostate surgery, faced challenges with pelvic floor strength. Through regular exercises and using a fitness tracker, John regained his strength and confidence. His story highlights the importance of perseverance and the effectiveness of tracking progress.

3. Samantha's Improvement in Sexual Health: Samantha, a 38-year-old woman, wanted to enhance her sexual health. By setting clear goals and using an exercise app, she noticed improved muscle tone and greater sexual satisfaction within a few months. Samantha's story emphasizes the positive impact pelvic floor exercises can have on overall well-being.

II. Lessons Learned from Others:

1. Consistency is Key: One common lesson from these success stories is the importance of consistency. Regular exercise, even if it's just a few minutes a day, leads to significant improvements over time.

2. Be Patient: Progress can be slow, and it's important to be patient. Tracking small improvements helps maintain motivation and highlights that you're on the right path.

3. Utilize Resources: Don't hesitate to use tools and resources available to you. Whether it's apps, fitness trackers, or support groups, these tools can make your journey easier and more effective.

4. Seek Support: Sharing your journey with others, whether it's through support groups or online communities, can provide encouragement and advice. Learning from others' experiences can offer new strategies and keep you motivated.

CONCLUSION

A. Recap of Key Points:

I. Summary of Benefits and Techniques:

Throughout this book, we've explored the critical role that pelvic floor exercises play in maintaining and enhancing overall health and well-being. The benefits are manifold: improved bladder and bowel control, reduced risk of pelvic organ prolapse, enhanced sexual function, and support for the core muscles that contribute to better posture and reduced back pain. These exercises can significantly enhance quality of life, offering both preventive and therapeutic advantages.

We delved into various techniques to strengthen and maintain the pelvic floor muscles. From basic Kegels to more advanced routines involving resistance training and integration with full-body exercises, each method offers unique benefits. We also covered essential practices such as diaphragmatic breathing, proper alignment, and the importance of consistency and mindfulness in your exercise regimen.

II. Encouragement to Maintain the Practice:

Establishing a regular routine of pelvic floor exercises is a commitment to long-term health. Like any fitness regimen, consistency is key. The techniques you've learned are tools that can provide lasting benefits if incorporated into your daily life. Remember, progress may be gradual, but the rewards are substantial. Be patient with yourself, listen to your body, and stay motivated by focusing on the positive changes you experience.

B. Resources and Further Reading:

I. Recommended Books and Articles:

1. "The Pelvic Floor Bible" by Jane Simpson – This comprehensive guide offers practical advice and detailed information on pelvic floor health, with exercises and real-life stories.

2. Heal Pelvic Pain" by Amy Stein – A must-read for anyone dealing with chronic pelvic pain, this book provides a holistic approach to treatment, including physical therapy exercises and lifestyle adjustments.

3. "Pelvic Power: Mind/Body Exercises for Strength, Flexibility, Posture, and Balance for Men and Women" by Eric N. Franklin – This book integrates mind-body exercises that enhance pelvic floor strength and overall body awareness.

4. Articles from the International Urogynecology Journal – For those interested in more scientific and medical perspectives, this journal offers peer-reviewed articles on the latest research in pelvic floor health.

II. Online Resources and Support Communities:

1. Pelvic Health Solutions (www.pelvichealthsolutions.ca) – This website offers a wealth of information, from exercise

videos to blog posts on various aspects of pelvic floor health.

2. The National Association for Continence (www.nafc.org) – A valuable resource for individuals dealing with incontinence issues, offering educational materials and support networks.

3. Pelvic Floor First (www.pelvicfloorfirst.org.au) – An initiative by the Continence Foundation of Australia, this site provides practical tips, exercise guides, and videos to help you maintain pelvic floor health.

4. Online Support Communities– Platforms like Reddit (e.g., r/PelvicFloor), health forums, and Facebook groups offer support and advice from fellow individuals working on their pelvic floor health. Engaging with these communities can provide motivation, shared experiences, and tips from people with similar journeys.

Your journey to pelvic floor health is a personal and empowering one. By integrating the exercises and techniques outlined in this book into your daily routine, you are taking proactive steps toward improved health and well-being. Remember, the key to success is persistence and self-compassion. As you continue this journey, utilize the resources and communities available to you for ongoing support and motivation.

Thank you for embarking on this journey with me. Here's to a stronger, healthier you, empowered by the knowledge and practice of pelvic floor exercises.

THE END